40

Prayers for

Healthy Living

By D. Duane Engler

& Ryan Andrews

1 Corinthians 6:19-20

"Do you not know that your bodies are temples of the Holy Spirit, who is in you, whom you have received from God? You are not your own; you were bought at a price. Therefore honor God with your bodies." NIV

"Haven't you yet learned that your body is the home of the Holy Spirit God gave you, and that He lives within you? Your own body does not belong to you. For God has bought you with a great price. So use every part of your body to give glory back to God because He owns it." TLB

Other titles by D. Duane Engler

The Christian Revival Diet™ © *2013*

40 by 40: 40 Short Stories with Less Than 40 Words © *2013*

Numerous Titles in the 40 Prayers™ *Series* © *2013 and the 40 Christian Prayers*™ *Series*

40 Prayers and Proverbs™

40 Prayers and Psalms™

and beyond

Comfort and ease can be our downfall. The easy life will probably elude us because after Adam and Eve got booted from the Garden of Eden we were cursed to toil. God wanted us to work and not be on a perpetual vacation! We were made to strive, work, sweat, and serve.

When our needs are all met we can easily become lethargic. Our tastes can veer to a momentary satisfaction but not for the long term. May the Lord help us to turn from these ways. Our thinking can become jaded without self-control and waste can overflow in our abundance. May the Lord bless our thoughts to live better for Christ.

If you feel this way at all, prayer can help you turn your life over to Christ and healthy living. These prayers are here for you. We pray that they might help give you a breakthrough performance in your life for Christ.

To God be the glory,

D. Duane Engler
& Ryan Andrews

*P.S. Check out the additional bonus material on prayer at the end.

1

Clean Eating

Lord, You provide our sustenance, our food, and everything we need to live.
Please help us to eat clean and healthy items that our body naturally craves.
Not only that, please let us hunger and thirst for Your righteousness.
We lift this prayer up to You, Lord Jesus.

Deuteronomy 14:4

"There are animals you may eat: the ox, the sheep, the goat." NIV

"These are the animals that you may eat: the ox, the sheep, the goat." TLB

2
Discipline

Oh, Lord, You are my light.
Thank You for being the standard to live by.
Having willpower and discipline is challenging.
It's easy to say I don't have the time or energy or I'll do it tomorrow.
Please help me stay focused and motivated so that my mind and body can represent You.

Hebrews 12:11-12

"No discipline seems pleasant at the time, but painful. Later on, however, it produces a harvest of righteousness and peace for those who have been trained by it. Therefore, strengthen your feeble arms and weak knees." NIV

"Being punished isn't enjoyable while it is happening – it hurts! But afterwards we can see the result, a quiet growth in grace and character. So take a new grip with your tired hands, stand firm on your shaky legs." TLB

3
Obedience to God

Obedience can be difficult, especially when I read other books more than I read my Bible.
Please help me to learn from Your commands, Lord Jesus.
Please help me to live for You, no matter what I do.
I know doing what I want to do can risk consequences that I don't want.
When I am disobedient, please give me gentle nudges to bring me back to You, Lord Jesus.

Exodus 15:26

"He said, 'If you listen carefully to the Lord your God and do what is right in His eyes, if you pay attention to His commands and keep all His decrees, I will not bring on you and of the diseases I brought on the Egyptians, for I am the Lord, who heals you.'" NIV

"If you will listen to the voice of the Lord your God, and obey it, and do what is right, then I will not make you suffer the diseases I sent on the Egyptians, for I am the Lord who heals you.'" TLB

4

Keep Your Body Clean

Heavenly Father, let me have the strength to resist the temptation to consume unclean or unhealthy foods. My body is Your body, and I want it to be pure.

Isaiah 52:11

"Depart, depart, go out from there! Touch no unclean thing! Come out from it and be pure, you who carry the articles of the Lord's house." NIV

"Go now, leave your bonds and slavery. Put Babylon and all it represents far behind you – it is unclean to you. You are the holy people of the lord; purify yourselves, all you who carry home the vessels of the Lord." TLB

5

Eat at Regular Intervals

Jesus, I sometimes struggle with self-control.
Please help me eat at the proper time and for the right reasons.
Let me stop mindless eating, but rather eat so I am strong to serve You.
Help the fuel you provide nourish me.
When I stray from the noble path, please bring me back to healthy living with You.

Ecclesiastes 10:17

"Blessed is the land whose kind is of noble birth and whose princes eat at a proper time – for strength and not for drunkenness." NIV

"Happy is the land whose king is a nobleman and whose leaders work hard before they feast and drink, and then only to strengthen themselves for the tasks ahead!" TLB

6

Eat for Nourishment

Lord, help me to control my appetite and mood.
Please give me the strength to limit foods that alter my mind and body from my mission.
You are the Almighty, and I want to live for You!
I do not want to be a slave to addictive foods.

Proverbs 25: 16, 27

"If you find honey, eat just enough—too much of it, and you will vomit. It is not good to eat too much honey, nor is it honorable to search out matters that are too deep." NIV

"Do you like honey? Don't eat too much of it, or it will make you sick! Just as it is harmful to eat too much honey, so also it is bad for men to think about all the honors they deserve!" TLB

7

Led Astray

Lord, while it might seem fun to use alcohol or chemicals to provide a temporary escape,
please let me be wise with my use of these things, so that I am not led astray and sin.
Please help me control myself so that nothing can master me.
Help me take time to really consider things that nourish me in mind, body, and spirit,
so that I could better serve You, Lord.
My goal is to be a good example of a Christian for You, Lord Jesus.

Proverbs 20:1

"Wine is a mocker and beer a brawler; whoever is led astray by them is not wise." NIV

*"Wine gives false courage; hard liquor leads to brawls; what fools men are to let it master them, making them reel
drunkenly down the street!" TLB*

8

My Body is a Temple

Lord, You have created all of us through You.
Show us the path to purity, righteousness, health, and cleanliness.
The purer we keep ourselves, the closer we remain to You.

1 Corinthians 6:19

"Do you not know that your bodies are temples of the Holy Spirit, who is in you, whom you have received from God? You are not your own;" NIV

"Haven't you yet learned that your body is the home of the Holy Spirit God gave you, and that He lives within you? Your own body does not belong to you. For God has bought you with a great price. So use every part of your body to give glory back to God because He owns it." TLB

9

Materialism

Lord, please fill me with renewal and refresh my soul with Your will.
Let the desires of this world fade away so I may be tuned directly into You.
Renew Your Holy Spirit within me, that I would make the most of each part of my day.
Forgive me when I have faltered, and help me be satisfied with only You, Lord Jesus.
This I pray.

Romans 12:2

"Do not conform to the pattern of this world, but be transformed by the renewing of your mind. Then you will be able to test and approve what God's will is—His good, pleasing and perfect will." NIV

"Don't copy the behavior and customs of this world, but be a new and different person with a fresh newness in all you do and think. Then you will learn from your own experience how His ways will really satisfy you." TLB

10

Strength

Lord, You showed what it means to be strong when You were being persecuted and on the cross.
It takes strength to live a healthy, spiritual, and faithful life.
Please help me remember that You are by my side.
Through this I can be strong and courageous, not scared or discouraged.

Joshua 1:9

"Have I not commanded you? Be strong and courageous. Do not be afraid; do not be discouraged, for the Lord your God will be with you wherever you go." NIV

"Yes, be bold and strong! Banish fear and doubt! For remember, the Lord your God is with you wherever you go." TLB

11
Live in Peace

Lord, please satisfy my soul.
Help the peace that transcends all understanding, Your peace, enter my heart.
Give me a longing for You.
Help my hunger and thirst be focused on You.
Help satisfaction and joy be in my heart, mind, and soul.
I pray for healthy living, quality rest, and Your comfort for me, my loved ones, other brothers and sisters in Christ,
and especially anyone who doesn't know You in their life.

Proverbs 14:30

"A heart at peace gives life to the body, but envy rots the bones." NIV

"A relaxed attitude lengthens a man's life; jealousy rots it away." TLB

12

Selflessness

Dear Jesus, my Savior, it's hard to put others before ourselves.
We forget You are the perfect example of being selfless and thinking of others first.
Please help me to live by your Word as You know best and are the ultimate role model.

Proverbs 3:7-8

"Do not be wise in your own eyes; fear the Lord and shun evil. This will bring health to your body and nourishment to your bones." NIV

"Don't be conceited, sure of your own wisdom. Instead, trust and reverence the Lord, and turn your back on evil; when you do that, then you will be given renewed health and vitality." TLB

13

Hope

Lord Jesus,
please grant me wisdom in thought, walk, word, and deed,
that I may know the right things to think, speak, and do.
If there is something that is not pleasing to You,
please help me to know where, when, and how to approach it, longing for Your word in everything.
Please renew my strength in You and help me to not grow weary, faint, or frustrated.
Help me to run, honoring You.

Isaiah 40:29-31

"He gives strength to the weary and increase the power of the weak. Even youths grow tired and weary, and young men stumble and fall; but those who hope in the Lord will renew their strength. They will soar on wings like eagles; they will run and not grow weary, they will walk and not be faint." NIV

"He gives power to the tired and worn out, and strength to the weak. Even the youths shall be exhausted, and the young men will all give up. But they that wait upon the Lord shall renew their strength. They shall mount up with wings like eagles; they shall run and not be weary; they shall walk and not faint." TLB

14

Perseverance

Heavenly Father, You are the All-powerful.
Life is tough. I know this.
But having You in my life is so great.
Talking to You is such a release and so comforting.
Please stay with me when things are tough, because then I can conquer anything.

Philippians 4:13

"I can do all this through him who gives me strength."

*"For I can do everything God asks me to with the help of
Christ who gives me the strength and power." TLB*

15

Endurance

Lord Jesus, my life is a marathon-not a sprint.
Sometime I feel like I've hit a wall and can't go on.
That wall is usually my own limitations and self-reliance.
Please help me to let go of my power and solely plug into Your awesome and wonderful strength.
I know You can carry me.   Help me to endure and remain pure.

Hebrews 12:1

"Therefore, since we are surrounded by such a great cloud of witnesses, let us throw off everything that hinders and the sin that so easily entangles. And let us run with perseverance the race marked out for us." NIV

"Since we have such a huge crowd of men of faith watching us from the grandstands, let us strip off anything that slows us down or holds us back, and especially those sins that wrap themselves so tightly around our feet and trip us up; and let us run with patience the particular race that God has set before us." TLB

16

Humility

Father, we are often treated with arrogance and self-centeredness.
Your Word shows this way of treating others is wrong.
It isn't healthy for our relationships and can affect our health, too.
Remind me of the feelings that kind of treatment gave me if I am ever close to being arrogant
Please help me be humble when it's tempting to be boastful or self-centered.

James 4:6

"But he gives us more grace. That is why Scripture says: "God opposes the proud but shows favor to the humble."
NIV

But He gives us more and more strength to stand against all such evil longings. As the Scripture says, God gives
strength to the humble but sets himself against the proud and haughty." TLB

17

Know My Limits

Jesus, now that I know You and Your commands for my life, my conscience feels totally convicted.
Please help me to know the limits You've set before me.
Remind me, Lord, where I sin or where I have become weak for Your cause.
Keep the truth, Your truth, branded on my conscience.

Hebrews 10:26

*"If we deliberately keep on sinning after we have received the knowledge of the truth,
no sacrifice for sins is left." NIV*

*"If anyone sins deliberately by rejecting the Savior after knowing the truth of forgiveness,
this sin is not covered by Christ's death; there is no way to get rid of it." TLB*

18

Cheerfulness

Dear Lord, when I'm happy and cheerful I feel more motivated to live healthily.
It seems easier for You to shine through me.
I pray that when times are rough, stressful, or tiresome that I can remember that You are there for me.

Proverbs 15:30

"Light in a messenger's eyes brings joy to the heart, and good news gives health to the bones." NIV

"Pleasant sights and good reports give happiness and health." TLB

40 Prayers for Healthy Living
19
Mission Oriented

Lord, the fields are ripe with people in need of Your good news and love.
Remind me to not get caught up in myself but to reach out to others.
Lord, let me learn from those making a difference for Christ today.
Lord Jesus, help my cup overflow with all that You have provided for me.

Matthew 6:27

"Can any one of you by worrying add a single hour to your life?" NIV

"Will all your worries add a single moment to your life?" TLB

20

Accountability

Lord, through my faith in You, I have the strength to be the best <u>me</u> I can be.
It is so easy to deviate from the life You would like me to live, but I know You have high expectations of me.
I want nothing more than to please You,
so I pray that You continue to guide me in the direction You would like me to go.

Ecclesiastes 4:9-10

"Two are better than one, because they have a good return for their labor: If either of them falls down, one can help the other up. But pity anyone who falls and has no one to help them up." NIV

"Two can accomplish more than twice as much as one, for the results can be much better. If one falls, the other pulls him up; but if a man falls when he is alone, he's in trouble." TLB

21

Positivity

As a parent,
strengthen me, Lord,
so I can accept the position of authority with reverence for You.
Help me to do my best while instructing this little one.
Remind me that I don't need to be liked
as long as I am truly working in Your will.
My role as a loving parent must be in line with Your direction.
Give me a strong desire to please You, Lord.

3 John 1:2

"Dear friend, I pray that you may enjoy good health and that all may go well with you, even as your soul is getting along well." NIV

"Dear friend, I am praying that all is well with you and that your body is as health as I know your soul is." TLB

22

Faith

Father, with You nothing is impossible.
When things get challenging I begin to question my ability to accomplish my goals or tasks.
Take away my doubts, Lord; instead let me focus on doing my best for You.
My faith in You will carry me through the good and the bad.

Matthew 21:22

"If you believe, you will receive whatever you ask for in prayer." NIV

"You can get anything – anything you ask for in prayer – if you believe." TLB

23
Unconditional Love

Jesus, let me love others unconditionally, remembering all the grace You give me.
Let me not make my health become an idol.
Help me to serve and love others.
Let me have a genuine faith and love that connects with others.
I lift this prayer up earnestly, as this is probably my greatest sin.

Romans 12:9-10

"Love must be sincere. Hate what is evil; cling to what is good. Be devoted to one another in love. Honor one another above yourselves." NIV

"Don't just pretend that you love others: really love them. Hate what is wrong. Stand on the side of the good. Love each other with brotherly affection and take delight in honoring each other." TLB

40 Prayers for Healthy Living
24

Inspiration

Father in Heaven, Your Word is so inspiring!
We often struggle to stay motivated whether it is to better our health, our education, or our faith.
We pray that Your Word continues to reach out to us.
Your Word, Lord, is and should be our source of inspiration.

2 Timothy 3:16

"All Scripture is God-breathed and is useful for teaching, rebuking, correcting, and training in righteousness." NIV

"The whole Bible was given to us by inspiration from God and is useful to teach us what is true and to make us realize what is wrong in our lives; it straightens us out and helps us do what is right." TLB

25
Everlasting Reward

Lord, help my determination be for the prize.
Help me to discern how to achieve that.
For the prize is eternal life! Praise God!
You died on the cross for my sins, so that I could have eternal life.
You've granted me this reward when I confessed and repented of my sins and turned my life over to You.
Please, Lord Jesus, help me use every ounce of my strength to follow You.
No matter what I do, I want to graciously and lovingly do my best, for Your glory.

1 Corinthians 9:24-27

"Do you not know that in a race all the runners run, but only one gets the prize? Run in such a way as to get the prize. Everyone who competes in the games goes into strict training. They do it to get a crown that will not last, but we do it to get a crown that will last forever. There I do not run like someone running aimlessly; I do not fight like a boxer beating the air. No, I strike a blow to my body and make it my slave so that after I have preached to others, I myself will not be disqualified for the prize." NIV

"In a race everyone runs, but only one person gets first prize. So run your race to win. To win the contest you must deny yourselves many things that would keep you from doing your best. An athlete goes to all this trouble just to win a blue ribbon or a silver cup, but we do it for a heavenly reward that never disappears. So I run straight to the goal with purpose in every step. I fight to win. I'm not just shadow-boxing or playing around. Like an athlete I punish my body, treating it roughly, training it to do what it should, not what it wants to. Otherwise I fear that after enlisting others for the race, I myself might be declared unfit and ordered to stand aside." TLB

26

Self-Control

Dear God, having self-control is of utmost importance for me when trying to stay healthy and fit.
Please help me stay committed to my goals
and help me to be a role model for my family and friends.

Proverbs 25:28

"Like a city whose walls are broken through is a person who lacks self-control." NIV

"A man without self-control is as defenseless as a city with broken-down walls." TLB

27

Willingness

Lord, help me to allow Your will to be done in my life.
Help me to trust You in everything.
I may not see what the outcome will be, but let me journey farther down the roads You want me on,
even if they are challenging.
Help my willingness to follow You be my guiding light and true north.

Proverbs 3:5-6

"Trust in the Lord with all your heart, and lean not on your own understanding; in all your ways submit to Him, and He will make your paths straight." NIV

"If you want favor with both God and man, and a reputation for good judgment and common sense, then trust the Lord completely; don't ever trust yourself. In everything you do, put God first, and He will direct you and crown your efforts with success." TLB

40 Prayers for Healthy Living

28

Failure

My past failures and regrets seem to linger in my mind, Lord.
These failures often stem from times I strayed from healthy nutrition and exercise.
I pray that You will continually remind me that life is a journey.
If I fall I can get back up!
If I eat poorly at one meal, I can make up for it at the next by choosing clean, healthy foods.
If I miss my workout one day, I can make sure I get out for a leisurely walk
with a family member or friend.
Thank You, Lord, for new beginnings!

Isaiah 43:18

"Forget the former things; do not dwell on the past." NIV

"But forget all that – it is nothing compared to what I'm going to do!" TLB

29

Gratitude

Lord, I sometimes have wrong expectations and compare myself to others.
I may feel like I'm not as in shape or can't participate at the level of the other person.
Please forgive me for my wrong attitude and ungrateful selfishness.
I know I have not appreciated everything that You have given me.
Help me to give thanks in everything, Lord Jesus, the good times and the bad.

1 Thessalonians 5:16-18

"Rejoice always, pray continually, give thanks in all circumstances for this is God's will for you in Christ Jesus."
NIV

"Always be joyful. Always keep on praying. No matter what happens, always be thankful, for this is God's will for you who belong to Christ Jesus." TLB

30

Consistency

Father, following Your commandments can be hard.
But I am thankful for Your path because it has taught me to stay consistent with Your Word.
I thank You for this as it has given me confidence in my health, relationships, and career.

1 Corinthians 15:58

"Therefore, my dear brothers and sisters, stand firm. Let nothing move you. Always give yourselves fully to the work of the Lord, because you know that your labor in the Lord is not in vain." NIV

"So, my dear brothers, since future victory is sure, be strong and steady, always abounding in the Lord's work, for you know that nothing you do for the Lord is ever wasted as it would be if there were no resurrection." TLB

31

Attitude

Lord, when times get tough, let me just remember who I am doing it for.
Let me then pray to You promptly and reach for Your strength.
I can then work mightily for You.
When I am deciding whether or not to do something a bit more challenging,
let me consider pushing myself a bit more.
This could be in my workout routine, in my shopping for food, in my service,
in my fellowship with other Christians, or in any other area of my life.
Let me champion my reliance on You as I strive to achieve.

Colossians 3:23

"Whatever you do, work at it with all your heart, as working for the Lord, not for human masters." NIV

"Work hard and cheerfully at all you do, just as though you were working for the Lord and not merely for your masters." TLB

32

Longevity

Lord, thank You for the gift of life.
We all want to live long and productive lives.
I pray that while I live on this earth I stay reminded that the values I hold provide me eternal life with You.
I also pray that I can maintain the health needed to spread Your word to others.

1 Timothy 4:8

"For physical training is of some value, but godliness has value for all things, holding promise for both the present life and the life to come." NIV

"Bodily exercise is all right, but spiritual exercise is much more important and is a tonic for all you do. So exercise yourself spiritually, and practice being a better Christian because that will help you not only now in this life, but in the next life too." TLB

33
Patience

Jesus, where in my life am I not patient?
Please point that out clearly, and let me find calmness in You.
Grant me the grace to realize this with others in my life as well.
Help me to look for the intended outcomes in their striving and not have such a critical spirit.
Lord, pain is only temporary, and the affliction You give me will strengthen me.
Please Lord, let me know where in my life I wimp out and help me to endure the affliction for Your glory.
Lord Jesus, prayer is powerful!
Please help me to be faithful in my prayer life.
Please guide me to communicate closely with You.

Romans 12:12

"Be joyful in hope, patient in affliction, and faithful in prayer." NIV

"Be glad for all God is planning for you. Be patient in trouble, and prayerful always." TLB

34

Forgiveness

Heavenly Father, thank You for forgiving me my sin.
You are the ultimate model of kindness, compassion, and forgiveness.
There are many times when I fail Your example and struggle to forgive someone for what they have said or done.
But knowing You has given me strength. Thank you for this comfort, Lord.
Lord, please also give me the strength to forgive myself.
It is hard to forgive others if I haven't set myself straight first.

Ephesians 4:32

"Be kind and compassionate to one another, forgiving each other, just as in Christ God forgave you." NIV

"Instead, be kind to each other, tenderhearted, forgiving one another, just as God has forgiven you because you belong to Christ." TLB

35

Physical Fitness

God, You have redeemed me to You.
God, You have forgiven me for my sins and unrighteous living.
Help me to spread that message of grace to others.
Help my physical and spiritual fitness be aligned fully with Your will.
Thank You, Lord Jesus, my wonderful Father in heaven.
Help me to make the most of the temple You have given me.
Help my steps, my words, my thoughts, and my desires all bring glory and praise to You.

1 Corinthians 3:17

"If anyone destroys God's temple, God will destroy that person; for God's temple is sacred, and you together are that temple." NIV

"If anyone defiles and spoils God's home, God will destroy him. For God's home is holy and clean, and you are that home." TLB

40 Prayers for Healthy Living

36

Rest and Recovery

Lord, it is easy for us to GO! GO! GO!
It is much harder to take the time to properly rest and rejuvenate.
Your Word shows us the importance of resting and recollecting on what we are doing.
Please help me set aside time every week to rest and refresh my mind and body
so that I can continue to do Your work.

Genesis 2:3

"Then God blessed the seventh day and made it holy, because on it he rested from all the work of creating that he had done." NIV

"And God blessed the seventh day and declared it holy, because it was the day when He ceased this work of creation." TLB

37

Stress

Lord, You created my muscles to be broken down to become stronger.
I see the parallel in my life in the times You have gifted me with stress.
It was really a time that You were breaking me down to make me stronger.
The stress You've given to me is enough for me to endure.
Help me to realize as I am going through it that it will make me a better follower of You!
I love You, Lord Jesus!

Philippians 4:6

"Do not be anxious about anything, but in every situation, by prayer and petition, with thanksgiving, present your requests to God."
NIV

"Don't worry about anything; instead, pray about everything; tell God your needs, and don't forget to thank Him for His answers." TLB

38

Confidence

Oh, Lord, You are perfect.
One of my biggest struggles is believing in my own ability.
Thank You for showing me in Your Word that You are with me.
Please lift me up and give me the strength to carry out Your will.

Isaiah 41:10

"So do not fear, for I am with you; do not be dismayed, for I am your God. I will strengthen you and help you; I will uphold you with my righteous right hand." NIV

"Fear not, for I am with you. Do not be dismayed. I am your God. I will strengthen you; I will help you; I will uphold you with my victorious right hand." TLB

39

Over-Indulgence

That extra serving of cake. That extra piece of pizza. Do I really need it?
Where is this temptation coming from?
It's truly coming from Satan.
He tempts me to overindulge and to yearn for a life of opulence.
He wants me to succumb to worldly pleasures and gratification.
Please steer me clear from these temptations, and help me to flee when they come.
I know and am confident that You can deliver me, Lord Jesus. Please deliver me for eternity.

James 4:7

"Submit yourselves, then, to God. Resist the devil, and he will flee from you." NIV

"So give yourselves humble to God. Resist the devil and he will flee from you." TLB

40

Idolatry

Oh, Heavenly Father, You are the King! Everything I need is in You.
I see a lot of people idolizing celebrities and desiring the latest gadgets.
I am not totally immune, Lord. These desires try to pull me away from You, too.
I ask that You strengthen me to keep my values strong and focused on You, not consumed by material desires.

Colossians 3:2, 5

"Set your minds on things above, not on earthly things. Put to death, therefore, whatever belongs to your earthly nature: sexual immorality, impurity, lust, evil desires and greed, which is idolatry." NIV

"Let Heaven fill your thoughts; don't spend your time worrying about things down here." TLB

ABOUT THE AUTHORS

D. Duane Engler is a son, husband, father of three, and a friend.
He loves the Lord and strives to work to Jesus in all he does, although often falling short.

As a professional educator and speaker, D. Duane aims to help others live out Proverbs 4:26 as they consider the paths of their feet.

D. Duane resides in Edina, Minnesota, where he is working on his next book.

Ryan Andrews is a son, father, spouse, personal trainer, and firefighter. Ryan has a love for coaching and helping people succeed. He loves his family and strives to live Christian values as a role model for them.

His care and focus is on helping people discover areas of growth in their lives. With his Master's Degree in Exercise Science, Ryan takes a very analytical approach to each individual's training goals. He is always striving to help those who are training for eternity, as well.

May health, wellness, and God's strength fill your soul!

Author's Section on Prayer and the 40 Prayers™ Series:

What is Christian prayer?

Prayer is communication with God. Communicating with Him from our place of weakness, surrender, and vulnerability so He would work in our lives, strengthening us for the tasks He has called us to do. Prayer is asking Him for guidance and skills that would allow us to honor Him more. Prayer is thanksgiving,

Prayer has been defined as an utterance, fervent request, entreaty, devout petition, praise, thanks, beseech, or crave. While the Internet provides many definitions of prayer, let's review vital points about prayer from a Christian perspective.

Is Christian prayer cross-cultural?

Christian prayer is cross-cultural and universal. God put the need for prayer in everyone's heart. Open Christian prayer is easier is some countries than others. Prayer to Jesus Chris is: (1) open and non-restricted, (2) monitored, (3) hostile, or (4) restricted depending on the country you live in or visit.

A Christian organization (The Voice of the Martyrs at www.persecution.com) defines these categories:

"Monitored areas are being closely monitored by some Christian organizations because of a trend toward increased Christian persecution. Hostile includes nations or large areas of nations where governments consistently attempt to provide protection for the Christian populations but where Christians are routinely persecuted by family friends, neighbors or political groups because of their witness. Restricted includes countries where government-sanctioned circumstances or anti-Christian laws lead to Christians being harassed, imprisoned, killed or deprived of possessions or liberties because of their witnesses. This includes countries where government policy or practice prevents Christians from obtaining Bibles or other Christian literature."

The "God need" that is in our heart can only be filled by Him. Regardless of where you are or what country you are in, God knows your prayers even when prayer is not spoken out loud.

Who should pray?

Everyone. Christ calls us to pray to Him in all things for He is the way, the truth, and the life. No one comes to the Father except through Him. Start as early as possible praying with young children. The evil one knows he can tempt young children so you must start prayer early. You can even pray for children you want to have or the child that is in the womb.

Does God answer every prayer?

Pray and meditate on these verses regarding answered prayer:

1 John 5:14-15 *"That is the confidence we have in approaching God: that if we ask anything according to his will, He hears us. And if we know that He hears us – whatever we ask – we know that we have what we asked of him."* NIV

John 15:16 *"You did not choose me, but I chose you and appointed you so that you might go and bear fruit – fruit that will last – and so that whatever you ask in my name the Father will give you."* NIV

Matthew 7:7 *"Ask and it will be given to you; seek and you will find; knock and the door will be opened to you."* NIV

Romans 8:28 *"And we know that in all things God works for the good of those who love him, who have been called according to his purpose."* NIV

Isaiah 59:2 *"But your iniquities have separated you from your God; your sins have hidden His face from you, so that He will not hear."* NIV

If we go to God, but we are not in a right place with Him, what shall we do?

Ask God to prepare your heart to receive His Word. Read your Bible. Confess your sins. Ask a pastor or friend to seek direction by praying with them to God.

Where and when can we pray?

Anywhere and anytime. You do not need to close your eyes or be on your knees. On the other hand, you can close your eyes throughout your prayer and spend the entire time on your knees. Prayer happens in your heart and your mind. Keep in constant communication with him formally each morning or night and informally throughout the day. He is always there waiting for you.

What should we pray about?

Anything. Talk to Jesus as you would a friend. Tell Him what is on your mind, what you are concerned about, what you need help with. Thank Him and honor Him every time you pray. Ask Him for guidance and direction. Pray for your family and loved ones. Pray for people you do not even know by name. Pray for things big and small.

If God has full control and knows how things will end up, why then do we still pray?

We pray because He told us to do it. In Matthew 7:7, we are told to ask, seek, and knock. It's that simple.

Matthew 7:7 *"Ask and it will be given to you; seek and you will find; knock and the door will be opened to you."* NIV

How should we pray?

Many people who pray use the acronym "ACTS". ACTS stands for Adoration, Confession, Thanksgiving, and Supplication (which is a way of asking God for something). Do not worry if you are not sure which category your prayer fits in to or the full meaning of supplication. The reality is that God honors any sincere prayer.

As I am not an English major please forgive any grammatical or syntax errors in the prayers. When you pray, God does not care about the grammar or structure of your prayer. He just wants your heart; please give it to Him.

What type of application can you take from the 40 Prayers™ Series?

Application questions surrounding prayers and Bible verses are the most fun as it convicts my soul. Conviction draws me closer to the peace of walking with Jesus Christ. Consider these questions when you pray and read Bible verses:

1. What did this scripture mean when it was written?
An application Bible may be helpful – you can buy online or in any Christian bookstore.

2. What does this scripture mean for me today?
Reflect on what comes to your mind or what you are convicted by the Holy Spirit.

3. How can I apply this scripture to my life?
What specifically is happening in your life where this scripture fits?

4. What should I start doing, stop doing, or change?
Is there anyone who God has put on my heart that I should share this with?

If you need additional prayer, help, or assistance where should you go or whom should you contact?

Your local church or a trusted ministry to your specific need is a good place to start for help and support. The issues you face will benefit greatly from prayer. At times greater professional, medical, pastoral, or other support may be needed. Make sure you honor and respect your body, and do not be afraid to ask for help,

Why the 40 Prayers™ Series?

The 40 Prayers™ Series is a simple focus of prayer and action. The format is a topic, heartfelt prayer, and supporting verse. The intention is to make the books easy to access and read, efficient to pray for anyone, anywhere, and anytime, and filled with meaningful application with a biblical grounding in Christ.

What is the focus of the 40 Prayers™ Series Ministry?

1. Spark a revival in the lives of people through prayer to Jesus Christ
2. Reach others with the message of Christ's redeeming sacrifice of dying on the cross for our sins

3. Explain how to be productive, intentional, and resourceful with the gifts God has given us
4. Understand the need for prayer in our world

40 Prayers™ Series was started after numerous prayers on direction and application of God's truth in our life and the reality of God's sovereignty. Forty (40) is significant in the Bible as a number that means complete or completion. With these prayers my hope is that you would begin, develop, or enhance your relationship with Jesus Christ.

With the desire to leave a legacy of prayer for my family and children, I decided to retain my prayers for them in a written format. When a friend suggested I memorialize these prayers, I decided to publish them. After my death, my children will realize how important prayer was in their father's life. Hopefully, more than my immediate family will benefit from this series. My prayer is that these books would inspire you to pray, to grasp God's unconditional love and underserving grace, to bring people to accept Jesus Christ as their Savior, and to encourage and comfort others in need.

Many times in speaking with people we say we will pray for them or we write this in a greeting card. We end up neglecting that prayer time because we forget or are too busy. The 40 Prayers™ Series is something tangible you can send a friend or family member during life's needs, challenges, and celebrations, always keeping the focus on prayer.

I see a need for spiritual revival in our hearts, families, communities, and our world. Revival starts with prayer. As God as our sovereign Lord, if enough people reach out to Him in prayer, who knows what the outcomes could be. But He knows!

What can you do to support the 40 Prayers™ Series?

If you feel compelled, write a review where you purchased the book or recommend the 40 Prayer Series to others. That would be very gracious. You can bless one of your friends or family members with a copy. The book may bring him or her one step closer to accepting Christ as Savior.

We appreciate your support and fellowship through this prayer ministry. If you are feeling led to translate a book into another language, please let me know as we are in need of translators to reach others around the world. If you have ideas to benefit others through the 40 Prayers Series ministry or to reach more people, please let us know.

Let's rock the world with prayer!

May you live your life as a prayer honoring Christ Jesus in everything you do.
To our precious Lord Jesus Christ is the glory!

Many blessings,

D. Duane Engler

James 1:2-12

"Consider it pure joy, my brothers and sisters, whenever you face trials of many kinds, [3] because you know that the testing of your faith produces perseverance. Let perseverance finish its work so that you may be mature and complete, not lacking anything. If any of you lacks wisdom, you should ask God, who gives generously to all without finding fault, and it will be given to you. But when you ask, you must believe and not doubt, because the one who doubts is like a wave of the sea, blown and tossed by the wind. That person should not expect to receive anything from the Lord. Such a person is double-minded and unstable in all they do.

Believers in humble circumstances ought to take pride in their high position. But the rich should take pride in their humiliation—since they will pass away like a wild flower. For the sun rises with scorching heat and withers the plant; its blossom falls and its beauty is destroyed. In the same way, the rich will fade away even while they go about their business.

Blessed is the one who perseveres under trial because, having stood the test, that person will receive the crown of life that the Lord has promised to those who love him." NIV